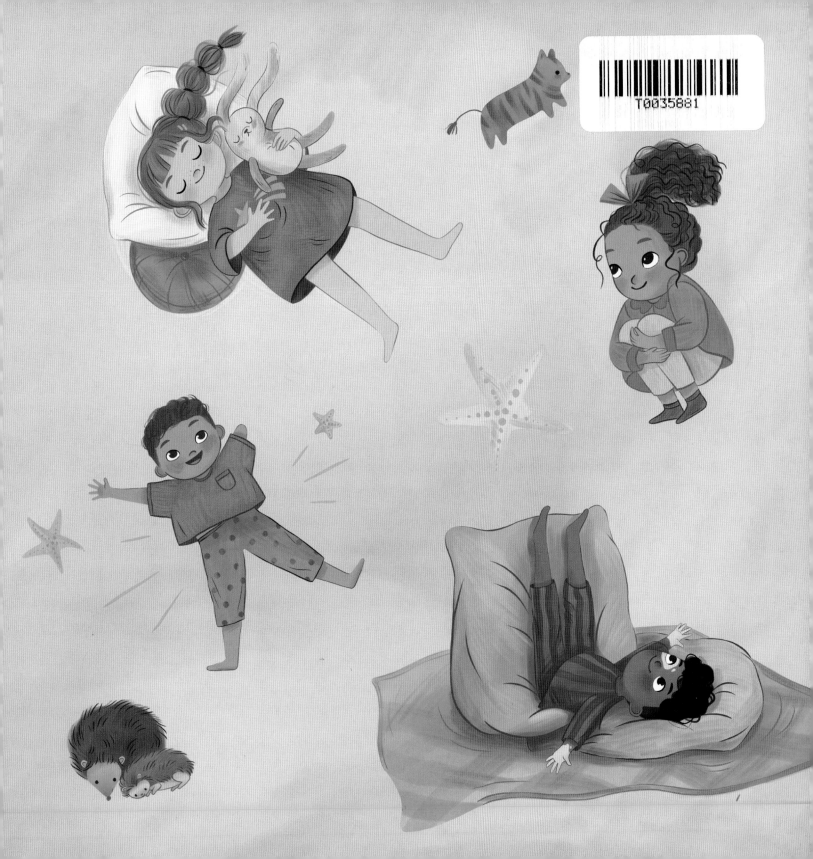

GOOD NIGHT, Body

FINDING CALM FROM HEAD TO TOE

BRITNEY WINN LEE

ILLUSTRATIONS BY

BORGHILD FALLBERG

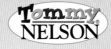

Tommy NELSON®

An Imprint of Thomas Nelson

For my own beloved body: home and conduit of eternal things.
—B.W.L.

To my lovely nieces and nephews.
—B.M.F.

Good Night, Body: Finding Calm from Head to Toe

© 2023 Britney Winn Lee

Tommy Nelson, PO Box 141000, Nashville, TN 37214

Published in Nashville, Tennessee, by Tommy Nelson. Tommy Nelson is an imprint of Thomas Nelson. Thomas Nelson is a registered trademark of HarperCollins Christian Publishing, Inc.

The Author is represented by Alive Literary Agency, www.aliveliterary.com.

Tommy Nelson titles may be purchased in bulk for educational, business, fundraising, or sales promotional use. For information, please e-mail SpecialMarkets@ThomasNelson.com.

ISBN 978-1-4002-3857-6 (audiobook)
ISBN 978-1-4002-3854-5 (eBook)
ISBN 978-1-4002-3849-1 (HC)

Illustrated by Borghild Fallberg

Library of Congress Cataloging-in-Publication Data
Names: Lee, Britney Winn, author. | Fallberg, Borghild Marie, illustrator.
Title: Good night, body : finding calm from head to toe / Britney Winn Lee; illustrations by Borghild Fallberg.
Description: Nashville, Tennessee : Thomas Nelson, 2023. | Audience: Ages 4–8 | Summary: "Bedtime can be full of big emotions for kids! Calm anxious, busy thoughts with this body scan meditation designed to prepare kids for sleep. This mindfulness practice will help children let go of worries, stress, and excitement as they reach their arms like a telescope, let their mouths hang like a hammock, dance their fingers like wind chimes"–– Provided by publisher.
Identifiers: LCCN 2022031687 (print) | LCCN 2022031688 (ebook) | ISBN 9781400238576 (audiobook) | ISBN 9781400238491 (hc) | ISBN 9781400238545 (epub)
Subjects: LCSH: Calmness––Juvenile literature. | Emotions in children––Juvenile literature.
Classification: LCC BF575.C35 L44 2023 (print) | LCC BF575.C35 (ebook) | DDC 155.4/124––dc23/eng/20220729
LC record available at https://lccn.loc.gov/2022031687
LC ebook record available at https://lccn.loc.gov/2022031688

Printed in India

23 24 25 26 27 REP 10 9 8 7 6 5 4 3 2 1

Mfr: REP / Sonipat, India / January 2023 / PO #12122148

Note to Parents

Body scanning is a meditation practice that gradually brings awareness to different parts of the body so we can release tension, deepen our breaths, and notice pain that we may be holding on to. This book is designed to help children (and their grown-ups!) lovingly recognize the communication of their bodies and gently invite this part of themselves into rest at the end of the day.

While this body scan speaks to many potential parts of the body, I recognize and celebrate that little readers and listeners will come to these pages with wonderfully varying forms and functions. Please use the pieces that serve you and your people best!

I hope that *Good Night, Body* will offer your little ones an opportunity to reconnect with their true and precious homes—their bodies. This mindfulness will be an invaluable skill for all settings and seasons, ages and abilities. Thank you for the invitation to be part of that journey.

Britney Winn Lee

Hello, body. Hello, dear friend. We've been with each other all day, but sometimes I forget to notice you! Would you like to spend some time together before we fall asleep?

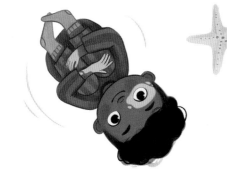

First, we need
to get out the last
wiggles bouncing around
inside. Curl up tight like a
hedgehog, then burst wide
open like a starfish.
Do it again!

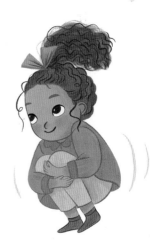

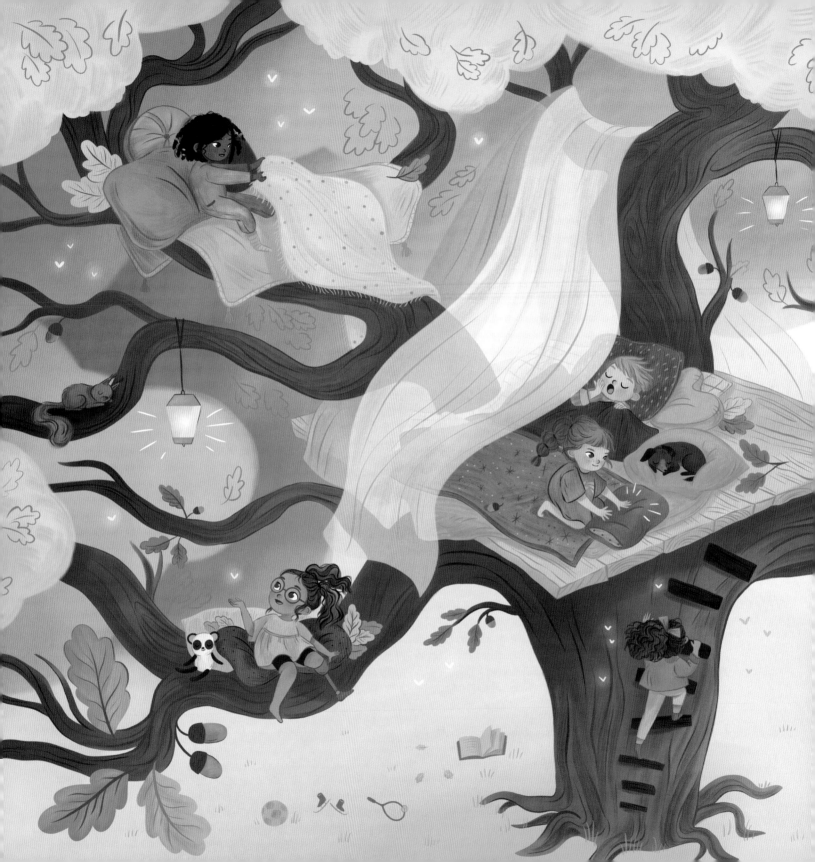

Now, let's climb into bed. Imagine it's a tree house where we can look down over the day. Snuggle into its safety and comfort as we find calm from head to toe.

Are you ready?
Take a big,
deep breath!

Hello, head. May you be light like a cloud. Follow the breeze, and float freely above the world.

Hello, mind. May you be playful like a puppy. Catch comforting thoughts, sailing by like bubbles, and gently blow the others away.

Hello, face.

May you be
slouchy like a
blanket. Smooth
any forehead
wrinkles, and fluff
out those cheeks.

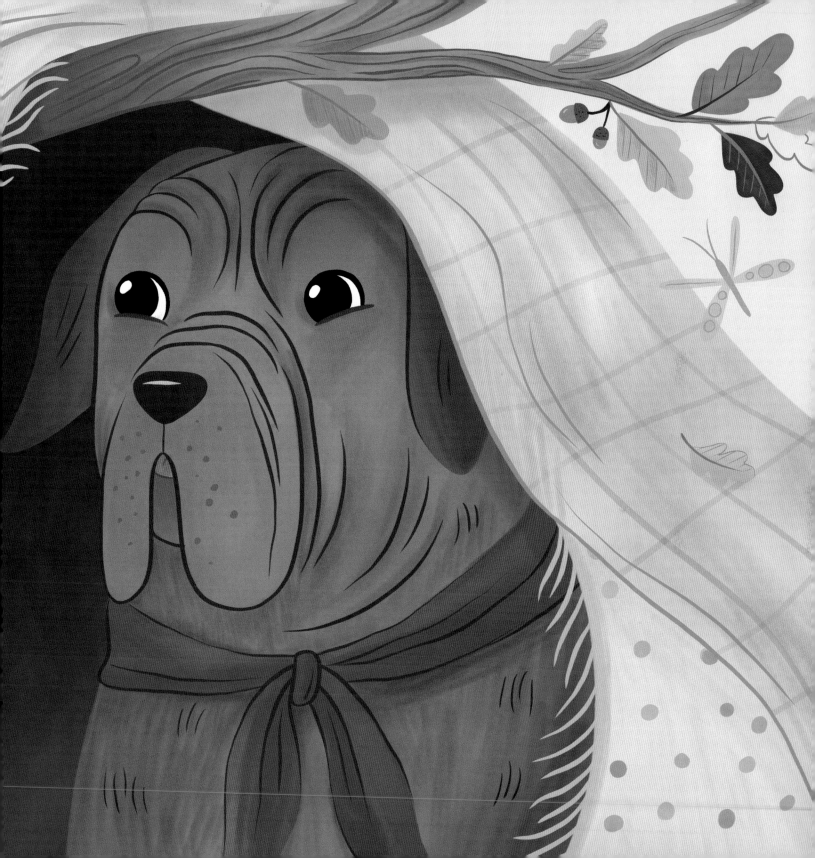

Hello, eyes. May you sink slowly like a sunset. Say "see you soon" to all the day's colors as you cozy into the dark.

Hello, mouth. May you hang loosely like a hammock. You do not have to smile or frown anymore today.

Hello, shoulders. May you be soft like dough. Rise way up high, then settle down into stillness.

Hello, arms. May you reach out like a telescope. **Stretch** toward the stars, and take up lots of space.

Hello, hands. May you be wide like sunflowers. Open to receive the warmth that life wants to give you.

Hello, fingers. May you dance like wind chimes. Flutter to the rhythm of your own special song.

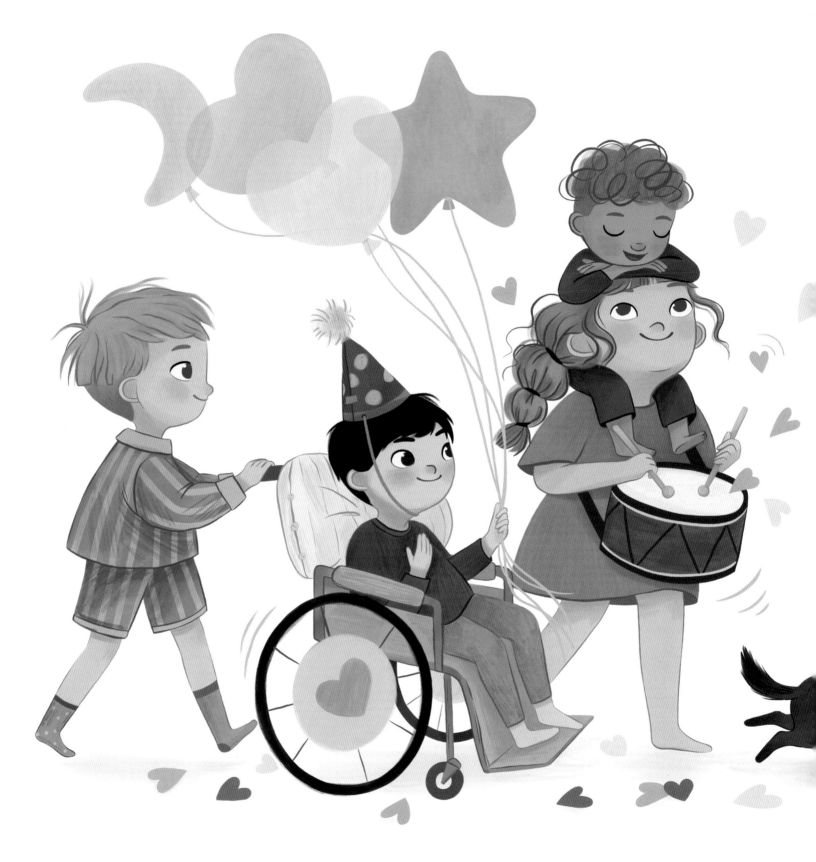

Hello, heart. May you feel steady like a faithful friend. Thump deep inside as if to say, "You're loved. You're loved."

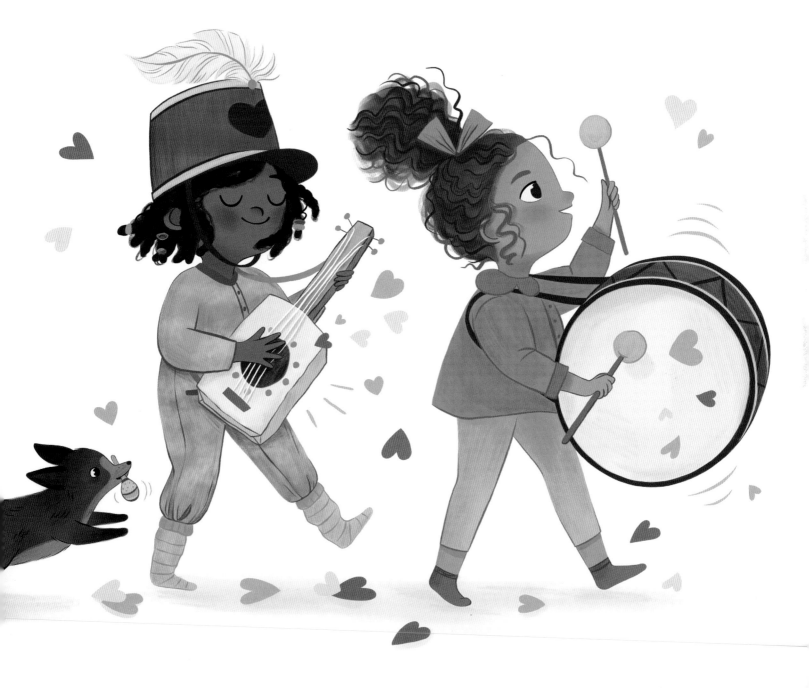

Hello, lungs. May you expand like balloons. Fill up with all the air the earth has gifted you.

Now release it like the breeze. Offer
breath back to trees and seeds as
a **thank-you** for their kindness.

Hello, belly. May you be comfy like a stuffed animal. Let me hold you close and pat you softly with care.

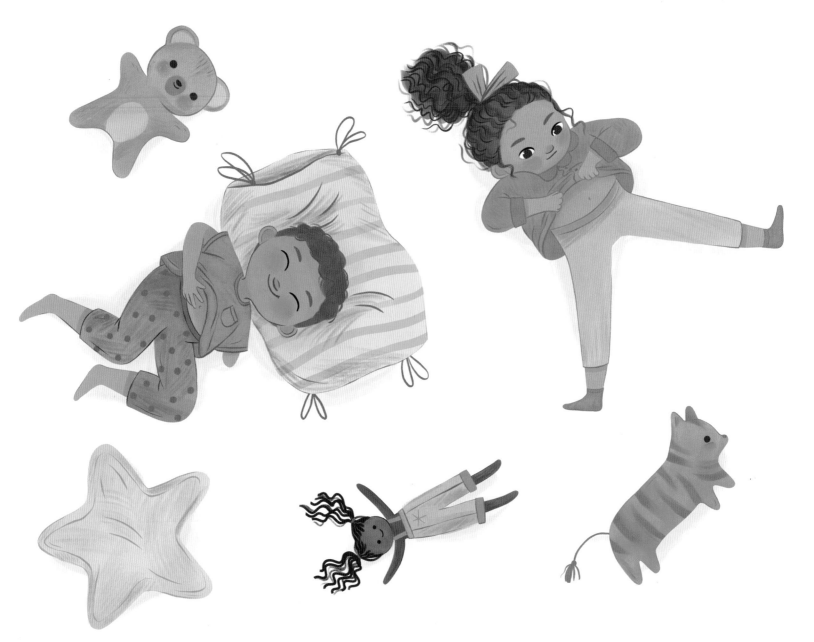

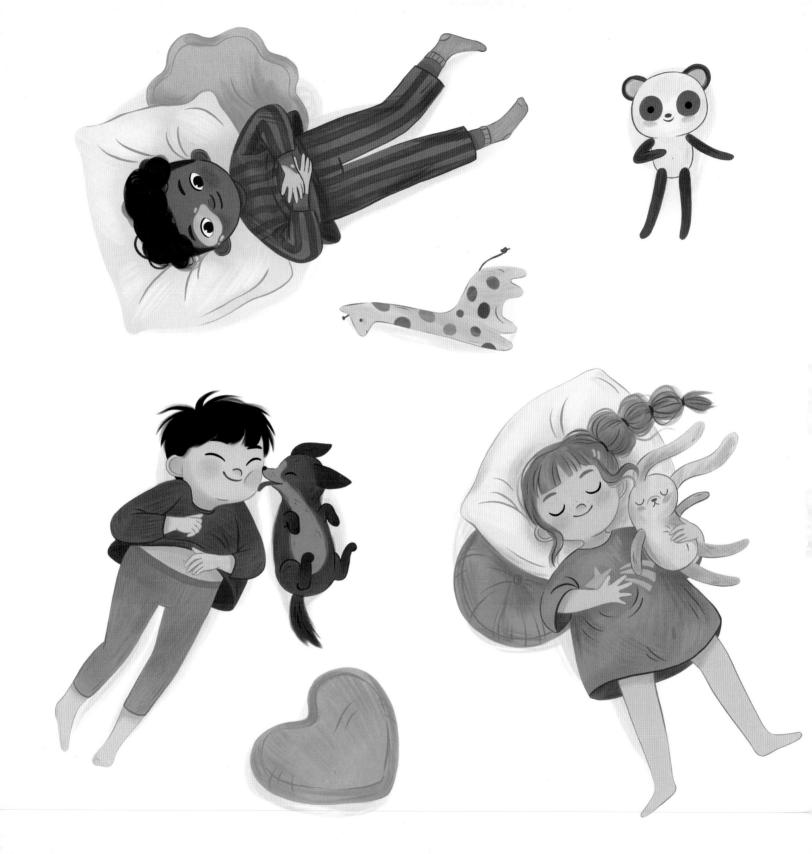

Hello, hips.

May you move like a seesaw.

Teeter out any tightness,

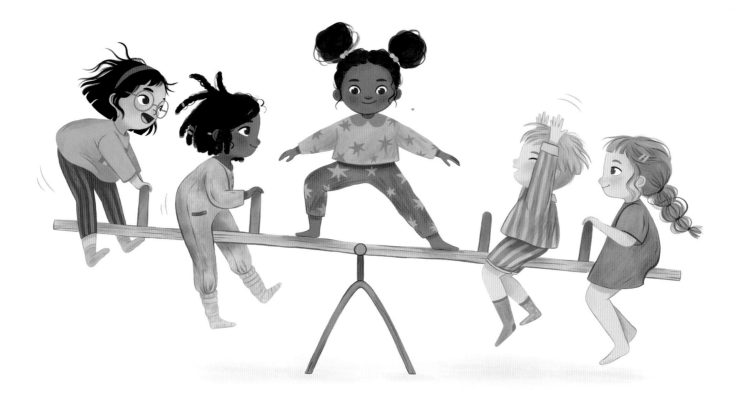

then come back into balance.

Hello, legs. May you stretch like a giraffe. Lengthen as far as you can go and then a little farther still.

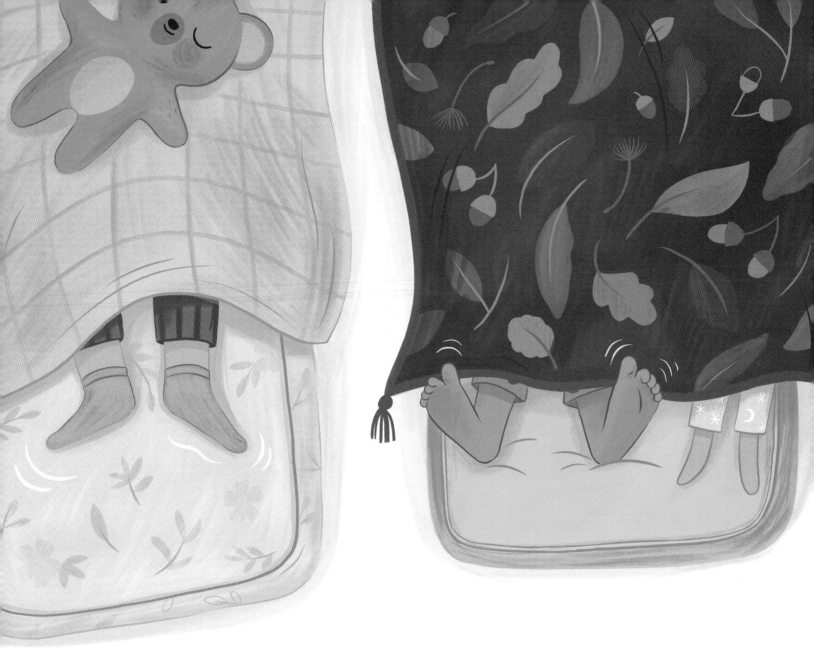

Hello, feet. May you rock like a chair on a porch. Move back and forth as if you are neighbors sharing a conversation.

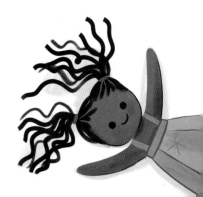

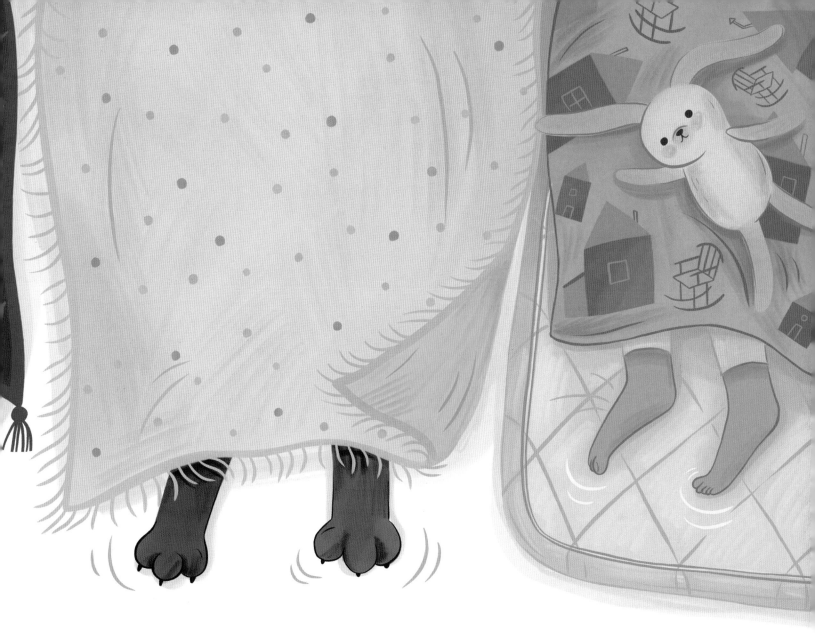

Hello, toes. May you be wiggly like worms. Squirm quickly and then slowly until I've felt each one of you.

Hello, body. Would you like to get some sleep now? I love to give you rest at the end of another day!

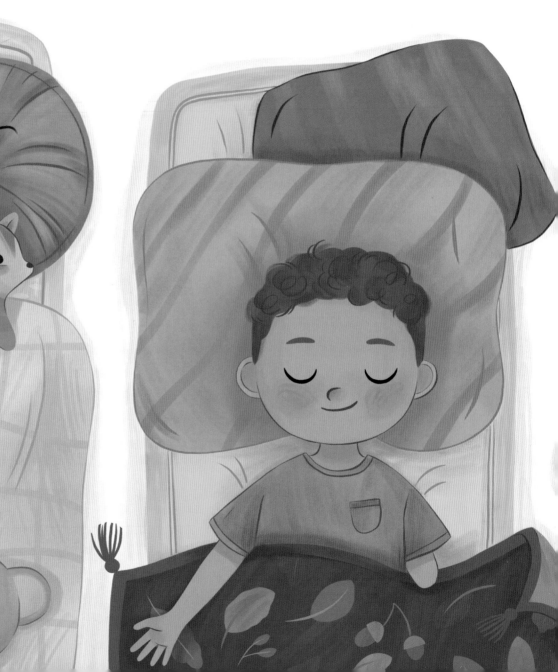

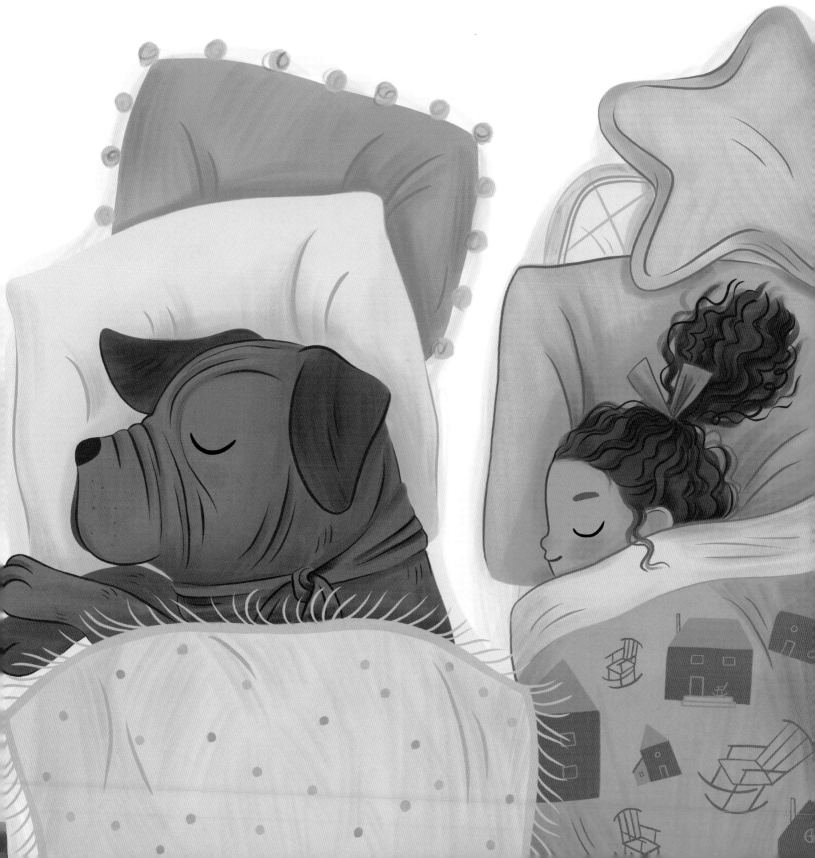

Good night, body.

Good night, dear friend.

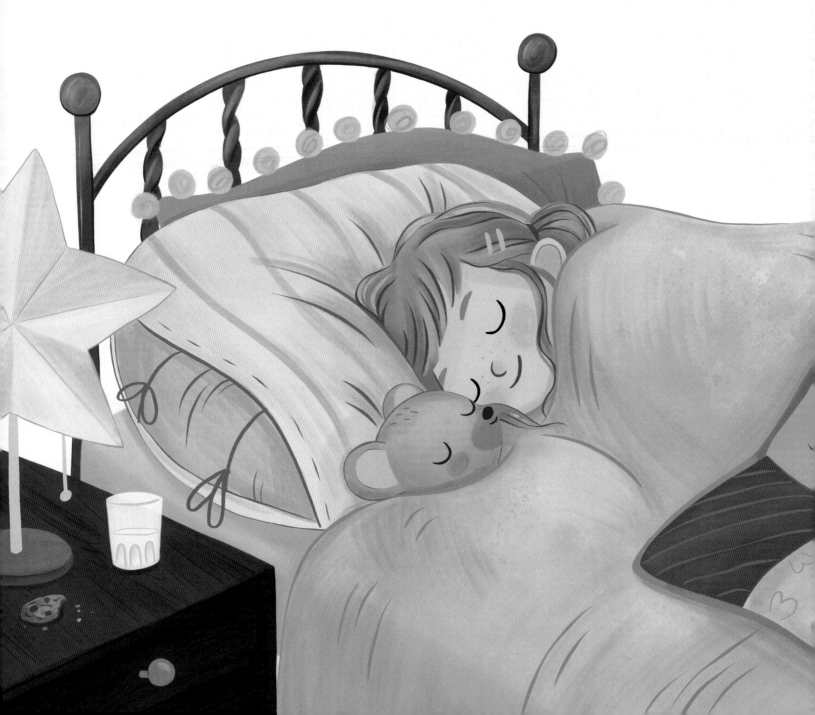

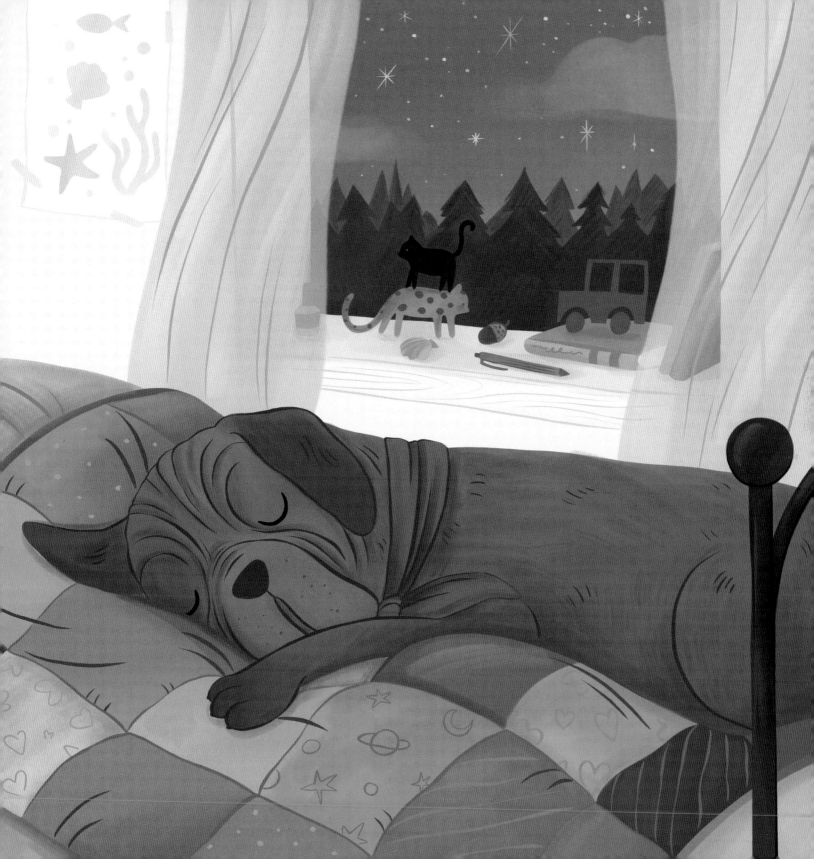

Thank you for being my home.

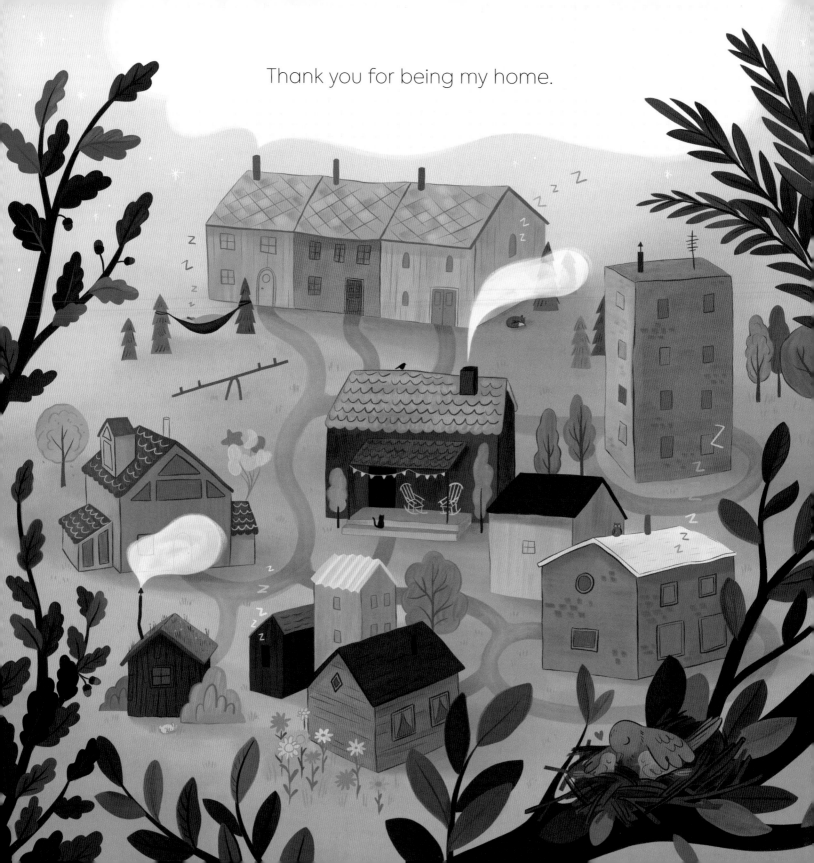

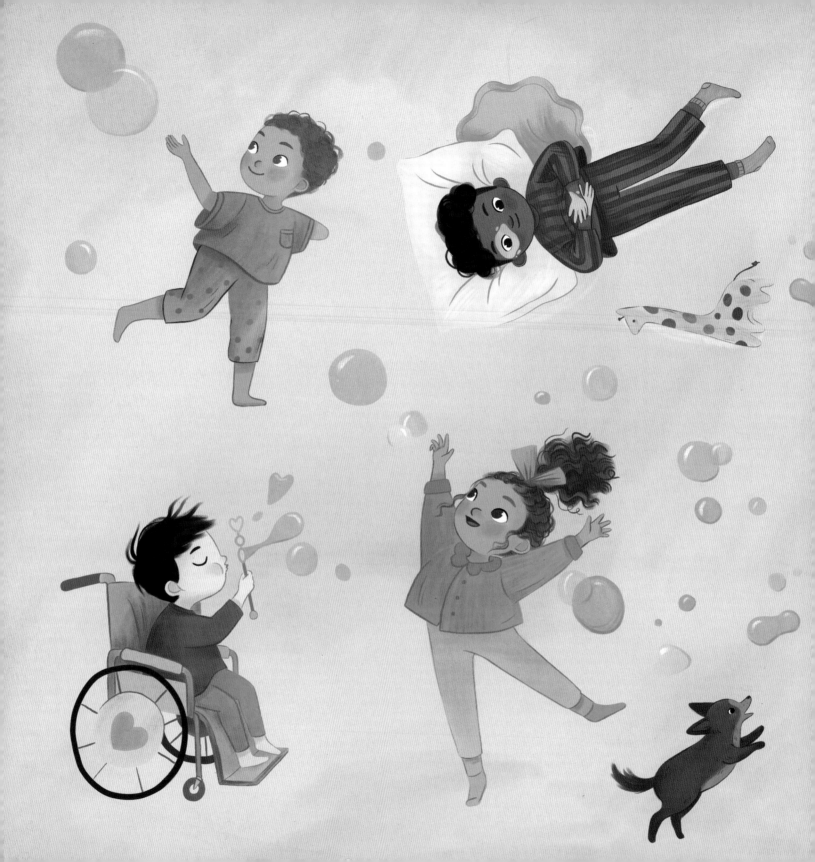